the *fourth*
trimester journal

Dear Hattie —
May this be a light
on the crooked path of
Motherhood!
Have courage.

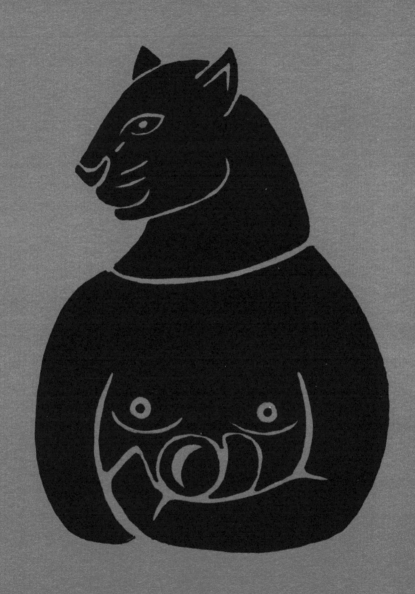

the *fourth* trimester journal

· · · · ·

Practices and Reflections to Honor Your Journey into Motherhood

KIMBERLY ANN JOHNSON

ILLUSTRATIONS BY JOANNA JOHNSON

SHAMBHALA

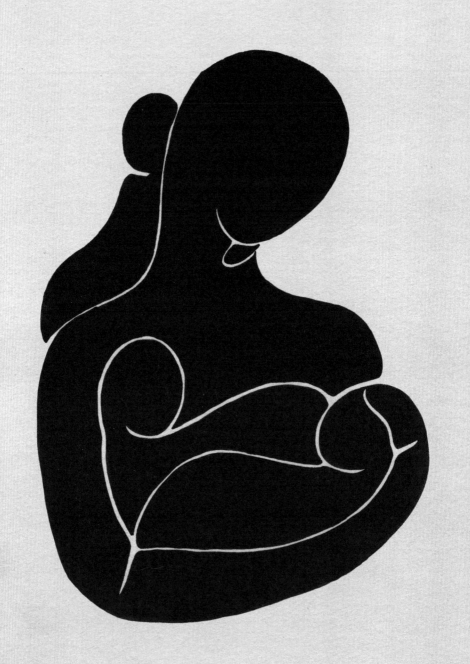

— Welcome —

This book is for all mothers. Even though it is called *The Fourth Trimester Journal*, there is no time limit on our evolution into motherhood.

Becoming a mother is radical, powerful, shocking, redemptive, and ripe for insights. Writing from thresholds is one of the most potent ways to capture who you are becoming as you live into each new phase of motherhood. There are lots of mother mysteries, and there is wisdom in them for you, your family, and our collective evolution.

This book is an invitation for you to anchor into the present moment; it's meant to spark inspiration and insight. There's no need to answer every question or follow every suggestion. Instead, take whatever moves you and follow the thread. During your days, if something comes to you, capture it here—there are many blank pages designed for just that purpose.

The journal includes an envelope, so that when you don't have the journal with you and you are inspired, you can slip in that napkin or paper scrap. Your partner or a birth attendant could hand you their version of your birth story and you can keep it here. You might print out some pictures and include them. You may come across a quote, a saying, or a poem that perfectly captures how you feel at this time.

There's no one right way or best way to mother. There's no one right way to use this journal. Make it your own.

Becoming a mother is a process of ongoing discovery. I hope that this journal is a trustworthy companion as you forge and walk this path of the mundane to the sacred all at the same time.

I designed this for you so that you have a place just for you. When I first became a mom, I had so many thoughts and emotions, and I kept wondering when I was going to be able to process them. This journal is a place of intimate connection, a place to be with yourself, or a sourcebook of reflection that you could potentially share with a friend and something that you can pass on as a legacy to your child.

Have courage!

Kimberly

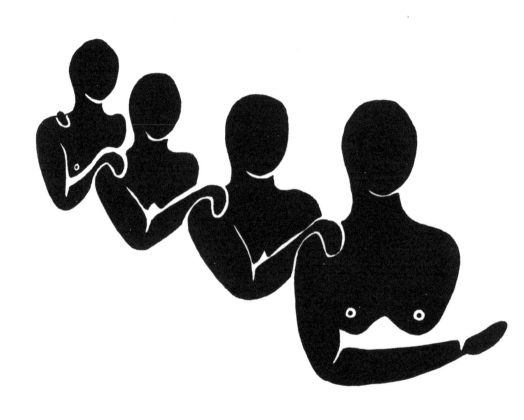

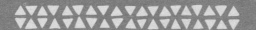

MotherNest

Motherhood is a mystery from conception through birth and forevermore. It is first nestled within the darkness and only slowly emerges into light. The first days, weeks, and even years of motherhood show us deeper layers of ourselves in profound and surprising ways. In this slow, unfolding process, there's a need for containment. Containment creates a felt sense of safety, where mother and child can find their rhythm together again and again. While we are in the process of healing and discovering the mother we are becoming, we need a MotherNest or sanctuary.

As mother with a baby, we are more sensitive and open than ever. This is a time when we need to feel protected and nurtured, pushing less and resting more, allowing for this great unfolding. Making your home into your version of a sanctuary, with spaciousness and safety, is one way that you can create a sense of harmony to settle into as you move through the unpredictability of the newness and the transitions. Our external world—our home, who's in it, the sounds we hear, the beauty around us—contributes to how safe we feel traversing our inner world. We need to be able to feel safe in our inner world—inside ourselves, and inside the nest we are building for our family. We build the nest, we live in the nest, and we are the nest.

Here is a simple body blessing that you can gift yourself anytime.

With loving attention, place your hands over the crown of your head and begin to slowly trace the contours of your body, moving from your head down to your feet. Let your hands linger in areas that need additional support. Feel the warmth of your skin. Attune to yourself as you do for your baby.

What does *MotherNest* mean for you right now?

• • • • •

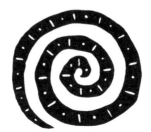

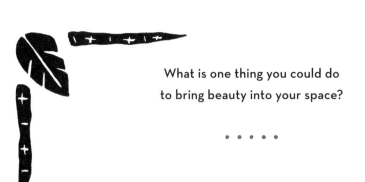

What is one thing you could do
to bring beauty into your space?

. . . . .

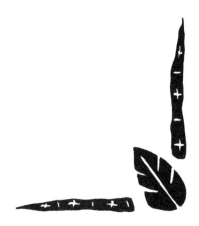

Do you feel as though you have or need protection?

. . . . .

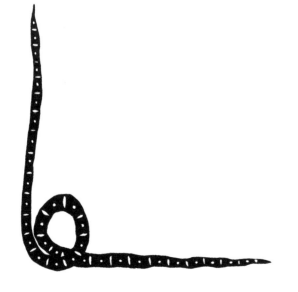

What are all the ways you are loving your baby right now?

. . . . .

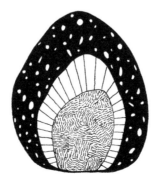

What is one small thing that you do for yourself,
or that others do for you, that makes you come more alive?

• • • • •

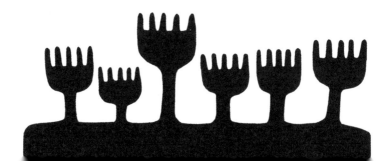

What music are you listening to?
What songs are you singing to your baby?

. . . . .

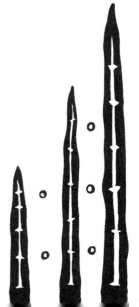

Everything that a new baby needs,
a new mother needs too.

What stands in your way of receiving? What is one thing you could ask to receive in the next week, even if you don't absolutely need it?

. . . . .

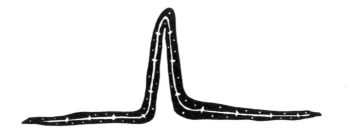

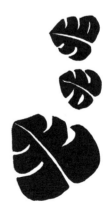

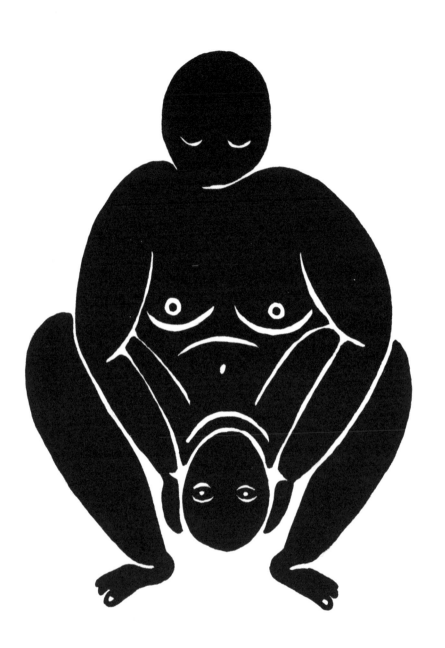

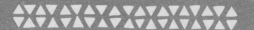

MotherBirth

—

When a baby is born, a mother is also born. We birth a baby and we birth ourselves anew. Giving birth is one of the biggest events in our lives besides our own birth and our own death. We are transformed and rearranged physically, emotionally, relationally, sexually, and spiritually—our MotherBirth. The story of the birth creates imprints for our relationships going forward. Most women can recall specific words, gestures, and dynamics many years later. These imprints hold deep truths and unsuspected keys to our maturation and development as women and mothers.

We get stretched to extremes and introduced to an even greater capacity to hold apparently contradictory opposites—gratitude and grief, joy and sadness, elation and despair. We can mine our birth stories for insights and gems that are gifts on our own path and gifts to our community as we honor our own MotherBirth.

Here is a short breathing practice to settle into your womb space.

Sit comfortably or lie down. Place both hands over your belly, below your navel. Let your fingertips rest softly on your pubic bone.

Inhale, let your breath settle deeper into your body. Exhale, soften the outer layers. Notice your belly pulsing with your breath.

Inhale, guiding your breath down toward your hands. Exhale, soften again toward your center. Continue this pattern for ten breaths or as long as it feels good.

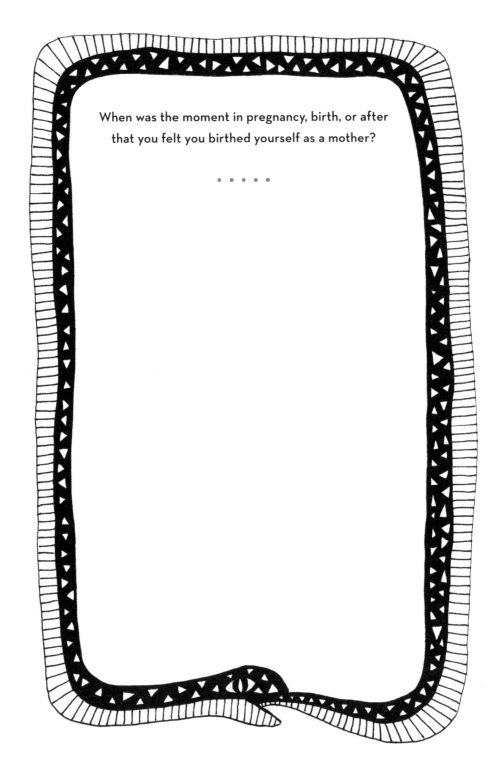

When was the moment in pregnancy, birth, or after
that you felt you birthed yourself as a mother?

. . . . .

Describe/draw a challenging moment in your birth.

· · · · ·

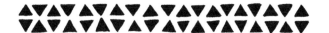

How did you get through the most difficult moments of your birth?
What resources, outer or inner, did you draw upon?

• • • • •

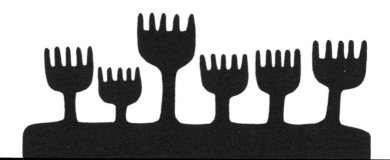

What did you do for yourself, or did someone else do for you,
that was helpful during your birth experience?

• • • • •

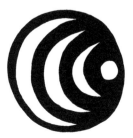

66

Birth is vast and multifaceted;
radiant and mysterious.
Birth contains multitudes,
and through her we birth
our multitudes.

99

—SARAH J. BUCKLEY, MD, from
Gentle Birth, Gentle Mothering: A Doctor's Guide to
Natural Childbirth and Gentle Early Parenting Choices

What was your favorite moment of the birth?

. . . . .

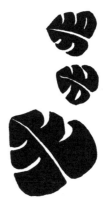

What is a lesson you learned from this birth
that you will always have with you?

• • • • •

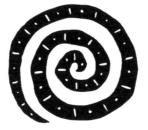

Create an invitation for the other people who were present
at the birth to share their experiences, and save them here.

. . . . .

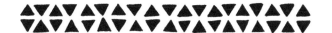

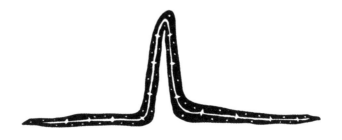

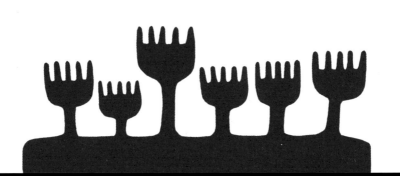

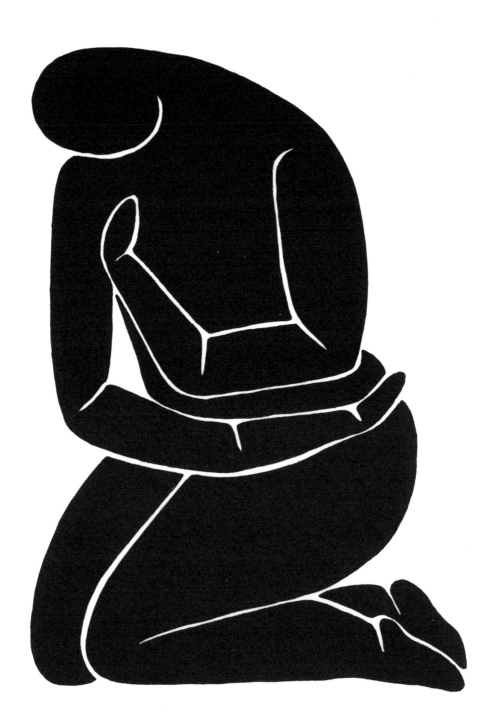

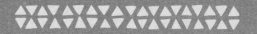

MotherBody

Coming back home to our body after birth is a process. Many of the physical changes are visible, like our profile that changes radically, growing and shrinking throughout pregnancy, birth, and the postpartum time. Many more changes in the MotherBody cannot be seen but are deeply felt. Our body shape-shifted to accommodate our growing baby, passed through the transformative portal of birth, and is now being called to reorganize at the same time as we get to know our new baby. As our baby grows, we too are growing into someone new. Feeling comfortable in our own skin can take time. It can be both confronting and liberating to meet ourselves again in our MotherBody. When we learn to rest now, we can return to activity honoring our body's present-moment needs. We can trust that our body is ever-changing, and over time, we will emerge with new strength and resilience.

Here is a simple breathing and mantra practice. Practice this for ten breath cycles, or more if it feels good.

Inhale: I am home.

Pause: This is home.

Exhale: I am at home in my body.

Pause: My body is my home.

How do you feel in your body right now? What feels new?

. . . . .

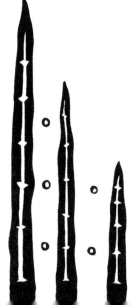

What part of your body do you absolutely love or are you in awe of?

• • • • •

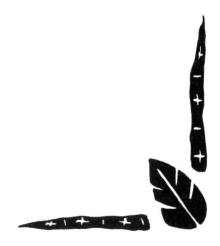

YIN	YANG
shadow side of the mountain	sunny side of the mountain
watery	fiery
dark	bright
cold	hot
slow	fast
nighttime	daytime
perineum	top of the head
feminine	masculine
mothers	children

Postpartum is a "yin" time. What is your relationship like to "yin"?

. . . . .

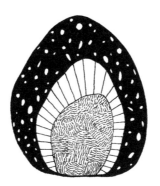

Write a letter to yourself from your pelvis.

What might your body be asking for that you may not be listening to?

· · · · ·

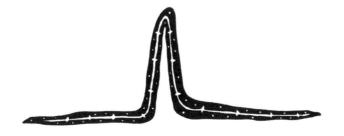

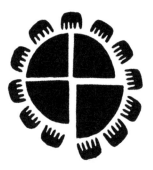

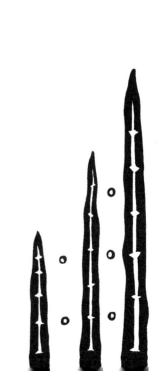

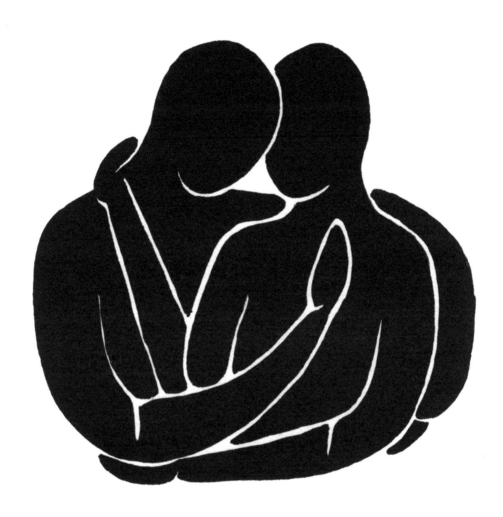

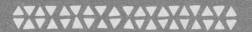

MotherLover

—

One becomes two. Or two becomes three. Or three becomes four. As our families continue to grow and change, so do our relationships and how we orient as MotherLover. The way that we can be a friend or a lover is different and evolving now. Sensuality and sexuality may be revealing itself to you in a new light. Our relationship to our body, touch, companionship, affection, attachment, sensuality, and masculine and feminine energies are all parts of what we lump into the category of sexuality. At this time, we have the chance to create a deeper level of intimacy with ourselves and our own erotic identity. Radical honesty and open imagination free of expectations can expand your palette of satisfying connection. This is a chance to deepen in intimacy with yourself as MotherLover and with your partner, if you have one.

Here is a mantra practice to guide your journey. Try repeating this to yourself or speaking it out loud.

I am worthy of love and attention.

I deserve to feel good.

My desire is important.

What is one thing you are holding back and keeping
a secret about your experience right now?

· · · · ·

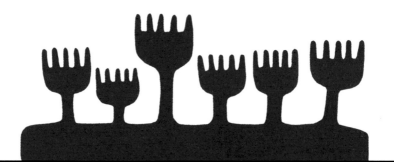

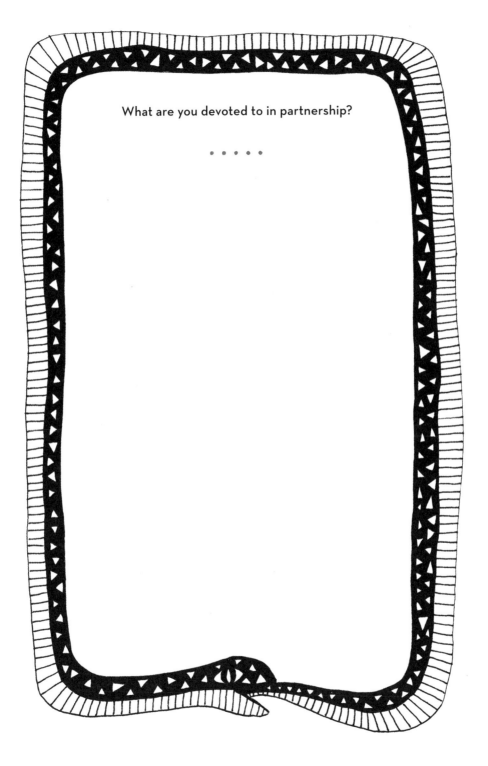

What are you devoted to in partnership?

· · · · ·

What do you need your partner to know about you right now?

. . . . .

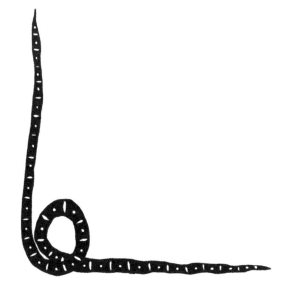

"

A woman who is directly and happily in contact with the true nature of her own sexuality is a woman who is genuinely in touch with her greatest power.

"

—UMA DINSMORE-TULI, from
Yoni Shakti: A Woman's Guide to Power and Freedom through Yoga and Tantra

What is the difference between sensual and sexual for you?

· · · · ·

sensual	sexual

What is the relationship between sexuality and spirituality in your life?

· · · · ·

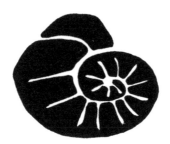

If you would like your spirituality and sexuality to feel more connected, what's one thing that you might explore?

. . . . .

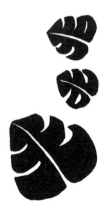

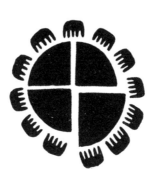

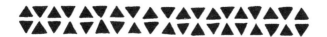

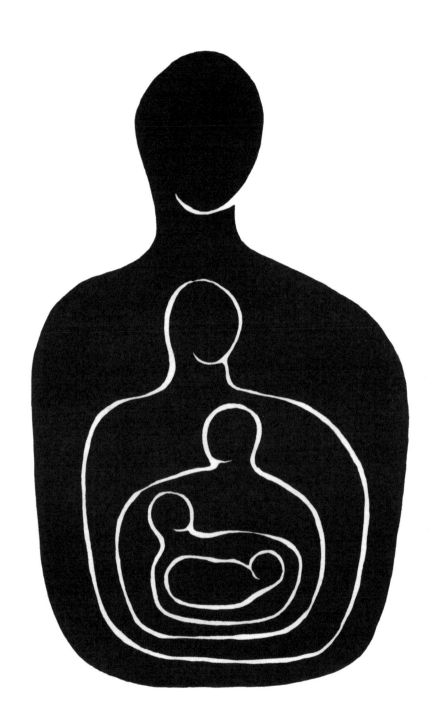

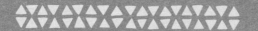

MotherSelf

New mothers need to be around other mothers. This is a time to come together—body to body. It's not just our baby that needs a mother right now. As a new mother, we too need to be mothered and mirrored as our MotherSelf. We need to feel that if we collapse, we will be caught. Calling in support in small ways will help you build a strong web that you can relax into. When we give birth to and raise a child, we re-experience ourselves at these younger ages and stages. We must re-mother ourselves, but we are meant to do that as we are mothered in community.

It's said that it takes a village to raise a child. That's true. It also takes a village to raise a mother. Most of us don't live in villages anymore, so we have to get creative about building them. Our happiness, well-being, and lifelong health depend on these human connections. A community of mothers helps us to see ourselves, to identify the qualities that we would like to embody, to give us relief in common difficulties, to be able to offer our gifts and receive the gifts of others. We want our MotherSelf to be seen and witnessed in our growth as mothers.

66

You are born with one mother,
but if you are lucky, you will have
more than one. And among them all,
you will find most of what you need.

99

—CLARISSA PINKOLA ESTÉS, PHD, from *Women Who Run
with the Wolves: Myths and Stories of the Wild Woman Archetype*

Envision yourself sitting in a circle of support, surrounded by other mothers and people who love you well. Notice how it feels to receive love and care in this way, being seen in your own mothering process.
Who is there with you in this circle?
Who feel like your people right now?

· · · · ·

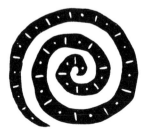

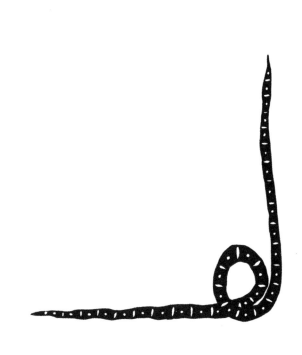

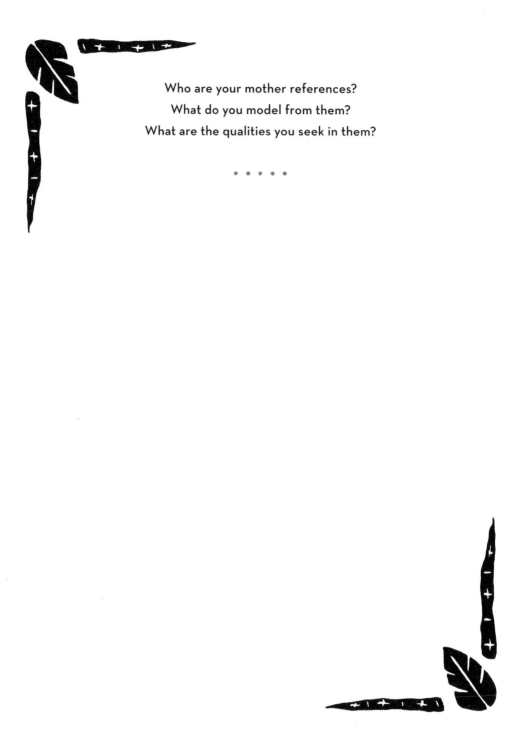

Who are your mother references?
What do you model from them?
What are the qualities you seek in them?

. . . . .

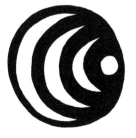

Who else mothers your child?
Who are *todas las madres* (all the other mothers) for them?

• • • • •

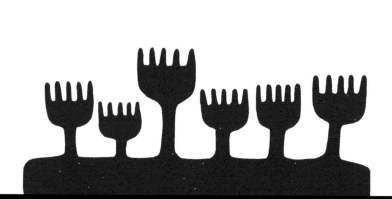

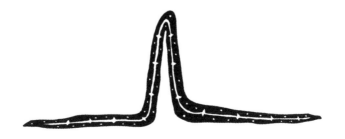

What kind of recognition do you want for how are you mothering?
What are the words you want to hear?

. . . . .

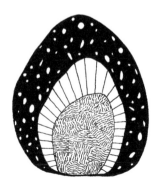

What experiences in your earlier life helped prepare you
for where you are right now in your journey?

• • • • •

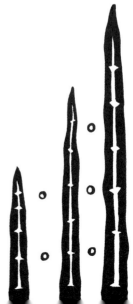

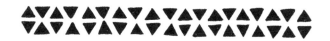

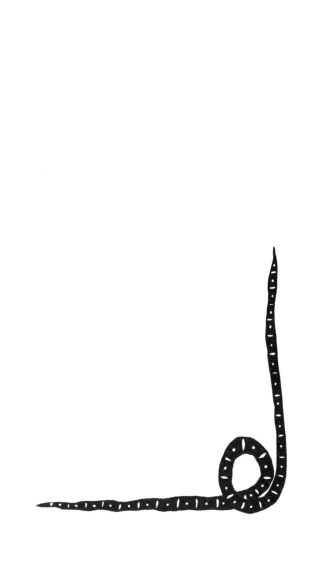

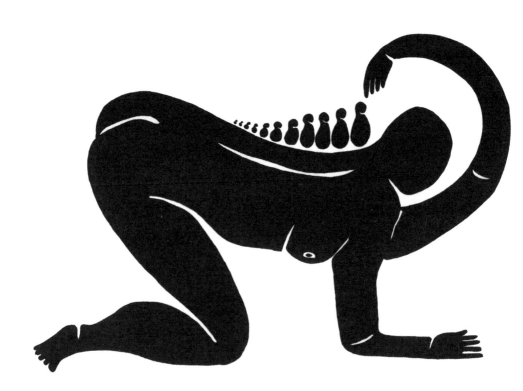

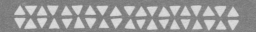

MotherLine

—

Every mother's journey is unique in its soul-stretching and strengthening capacity, yet we are not alone in the process. When the mother in you is activated, so is your MotherLine, our connection to our own mothers, grandmothers, and ancestral mothers through our matriline. Many of us have complicated relationships to our mothers. When we become mothers, our relationships to the women who mothered us will come to light in new ways. There is a great opportunity for healing, if that is what's called for. It can be both a reckoning and an awakening process, leaving us both rearranged, fortified, and full of gratitude for the path forward. We have the chance to leave behind what hasn't worked and consciously carry forward the emboldening strengths of our MotherLine.

Here is a visualization to feel the support of your MotherLine.

Sit comfortably or lie down if you can. Bring an image of your mother or a well-loved mother figure into your mind's eye. Try to capture her essence. Notice how you feel and let that seep into all the cells in your body. Now imagine any grandmother figures, again capturing their essences even if the images are unclear. Go back as far as you can in your MotherLine, perhaps capturing great-grandmothers or great-aunts. Notice the images or sensations that come. Surround yourself with the essences of your ancestors.

Know that there are those who come before you and those who will come after. Return to this at any time, if it feels useful.

What qualities of your mother and your grandmother do you absolutely want to carry forward to your own mothering?

· · · · ·

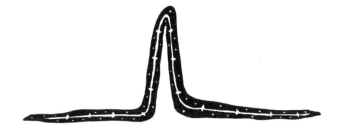

What does it mean for you to be mothering a daughter or a son?

• • • • •

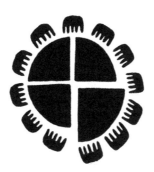

What were you taught is a "good mother"?

What are your expectations of a "good mother"?

· · · · ·

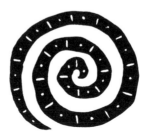

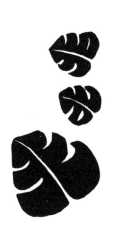

"

Our bodies and those of our daughters were created by a seamless web of nature and nurture, of biology informed by consciousness that we can trace back to the beginning of time. Thus, every daughter contains her mother and all the women who came before her. The unrealized dreams of our maternal ancestors are part of our heritage. Every woman who heals herself helps all the women who came before her and all those who will come after her.

"

—CHRISTIANE NORTHRUP, MD, from
Mother-Daughter Wisdom: Understanding the Crucial Link between Mothers, Daughters, and Health

What do you appreciate or understand about
your own mother now, that you didn't before?

. . . . .

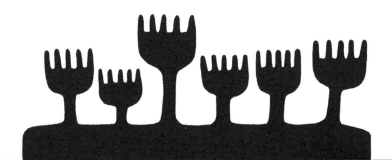

What patterns in your lineage are you committed to interrupting
and not carrying forward?

· · · · ·

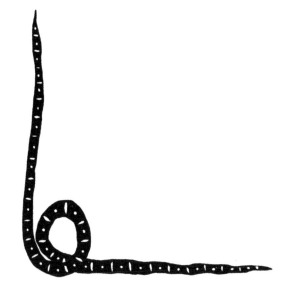

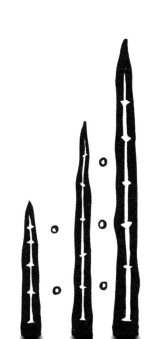

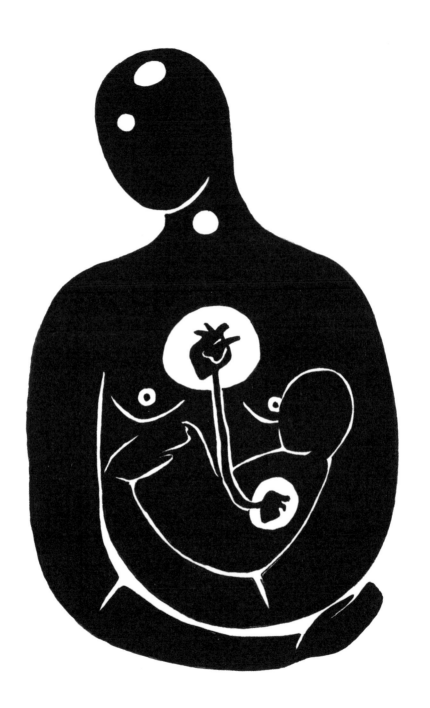

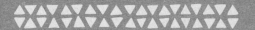

MotherBaby

—

In Swahili, the word *mamatoto* means "MotherBaby," describing the unit after a mother gives birth. The language reflects there is no dyad yet. As such, mother and baby exist only in relation to one another, and should not be treated as separate entities, let along separate words.

We are intricately linked with our baby, however we birth. Our bodies depend on each other for safety. Our nervous systems are still interwoven, even when our bodies are separate. We regulate each other. Early motherhood is the ultimate interdependence, unlike any other experience. This dance of interdependence and eventual differentiation is a process, unique to each mother and each baby. Our bodies may become more independent over time, yet the imprint of this essential oneness remains. We can find our own way and path through the maze of interdependence and independence by refining and listening to our intuition.

Here is a visualization you can use to explore coregulation and interdependence.

Imagine an egg-shaped energy field surrounding you, and one surrounding your baby. Notice the color of each as it takes form in your mind's eye. Envision both the merging and the separation of these two energy centers. Notice how you feel with the merging and how you feel with the separation.

"

A mother's body against a
child's body makes a place.
It says you are here. Without
this body, there is no place."

"

—**EVE ENSLER**, from
In the Body of the World

What has been your favorite part of feeding and nourishing your baby?
What has been your greatest challenge? How did you get through that?

. . . . .

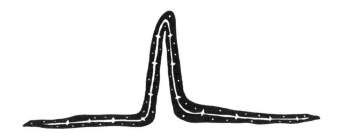

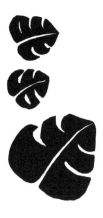

When do you feel most connected to your baby?

• • • • •

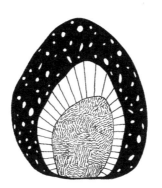

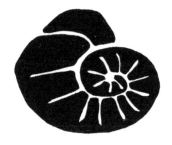

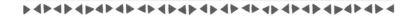

MEDITATION ON MOTHERHOOD

Crying breasts.
Crying baby.
Crying sky.

Milk,
tears,
rain

all moisten
and bring forth
what's coming

into being.
All we have to do
is the very next thing.

—**BROOKE MCNAMARA**, *Bury The Seed:*
Poems for Releasing More Life into You

What would your baby say is their favorite part of the day/night?
What is the hardest part of the day/night?

. . . . .

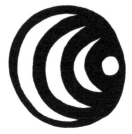

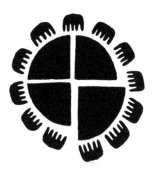

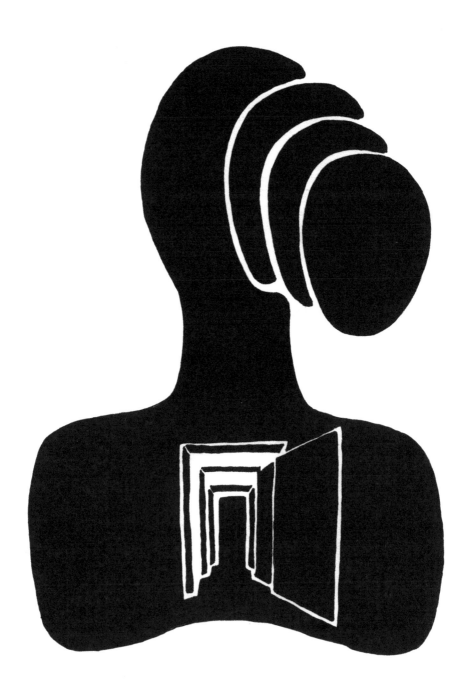

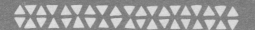

MotherCode

—

There's no one right way to mother. There is just becoming the mother we are. We discover the mother we are as we are learning to mother. It's a little like building a ship and sailing it at the same time. Sometimes the sea feels unfamiliar and stormy. Sometimes it feels like smooth sailing. Inevitably, whether stormy or smooth, the winds of change come and we are invited to meet ourselves and our child in new ways, again and again, as they grow and we grow. Finding our MotherCode requires that we consciously choose the pieces of our MotherLine that we want to carry forward as well as discard notions of how we think things should be in favor of how they actually are.

Here is a simple breathing practice to find your center.

If possible, stand with feet about hip-width apart. You can also do this seated. Gently rock forward and backward from heel to toe, or from front to back on your sit bones, until you feel comfortable yet steady and strong. Relax your gaze. Inhale; breathe down your center into your pelvis. Exhale; let the breath travel up the back of your spine to the crown of your head. Inhale, back down to your perineum, the breath washing over you like a cleansing rain. Exhale, the breath fortifying you as it reaches the crown of your head.

Continue for ten breath cycles or as long as it feels nourishing.

"

Taking care of a child is
like weaving a great tapestry;
it starts with a simple thread and,
through day-to-day tending
over a long period of time, evolves
into an intricate creation.

"

—TAMI LYNN KENT, from
*Mothering from Your Center: Tapping Your Body's
Natural Energy for Pregnancy, Birth, and Parenting*

What parts of mothering have surprised you?

· · · · ·

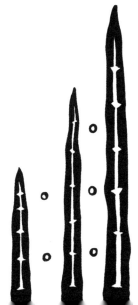

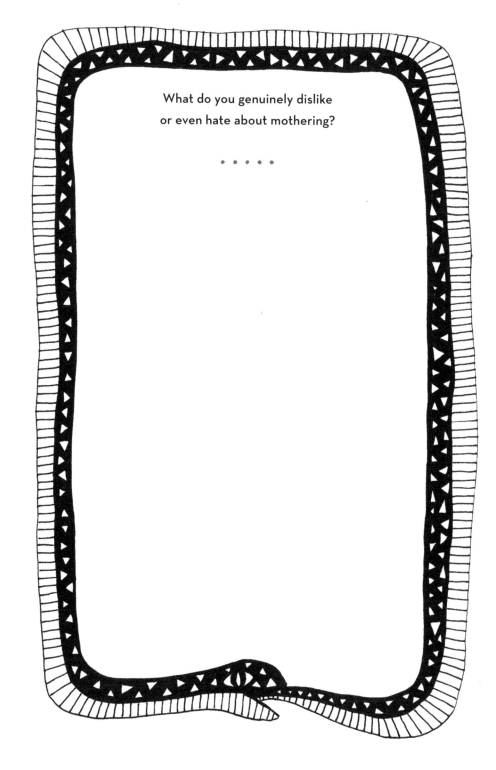

What do you genuinely dislike
or even hate about mothering?

· · · · ·

What is one part of mothering that has come easily to you?

· · · · ·

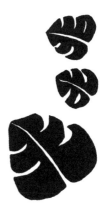

What have you had to give up in becoming a mother?

· · · · ·

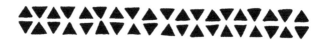

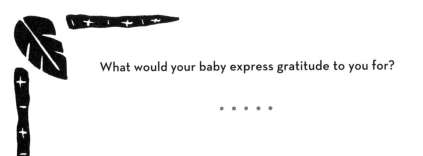

What would your baby express gratitude to you for?

. . . . .

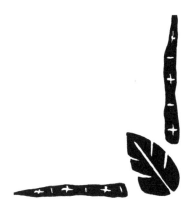

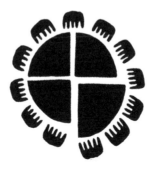

What are your highest values that you want to make sure
your child upholds or understands?

• • • • •

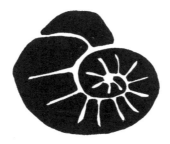

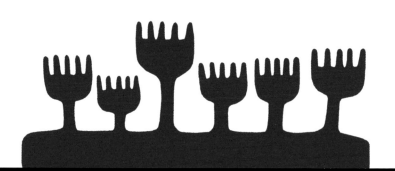

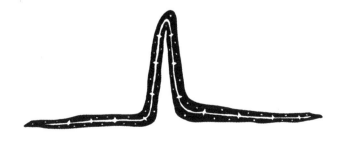

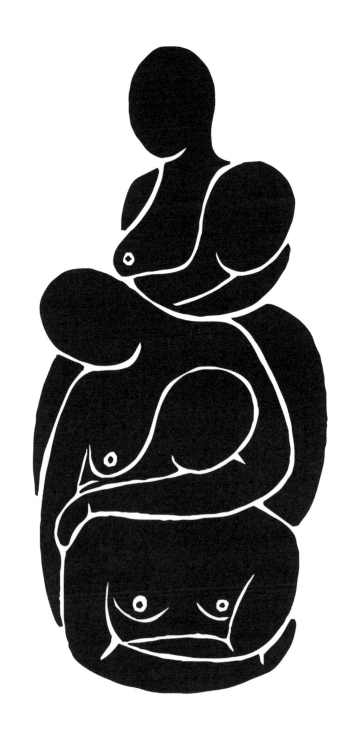

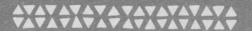

MotherLegacy

—

While the MotherCode practices involve looking back and discerning what to keep and discard, MotherLegacy is our unique future. It's easy for most of us to look back, it is more of a stretch to look ahead and consider what we would like to impart as our own MotherLegacy. We have a powerful opportunity, every day, to imagine the legacy we'd like to leave, even if we don't do it perfectly. Taking space to consider what we want our child to remember about who we are and who they are during this time creates the foundation for our MotherLegacy. We give our child a tremendous gift by letting our unique voice come through in our mothering. Discovering our MotherLegacy may take time, yet it's ultimately a reflection of our own true nature. Allow yourself to focus on what truly lights you up in mothering.

Here's a short guided meditation to sense into your MotherLegacy.

Sit comfortably in a space without distractions. Set a timer for as short as three minutes or as long as thirteen, depending on your needs. Hold this inquiry in your awareness:

What gift(s) will I leave my child?

You can state the inquiry out loud or imagine it in your mind's eye. Be with any thoughts, images, or sensations that arise. Let it have its own rhythm and timing. The breath can be your anchor point if needed.

When the time is up, note anything that stays with you.

On the opposite page, you will see four circles. The circle on the bottom is you. The circle above is your mother or a mother figure, and then above that are two circles for your maternal and paternal grandmothers or grandparent figures. Label the circles with their names and yours.

On the left half of each circle, place the qualities of your grandmothers that are negative or damaging, the things you don't like and would like to leave behind. On the right half of the circle, write down what you love about each of them. Do the same for your mother in the middle circle.

Then, come down to your circle. Fill your circle with the positive qualities from the right sides of the circles above, the things that you would like to pass on to your children. This is your beautiful family lineage.

On the next page, there are a few questions about this exercise to consider.

• • • • •

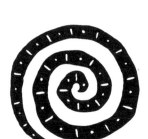

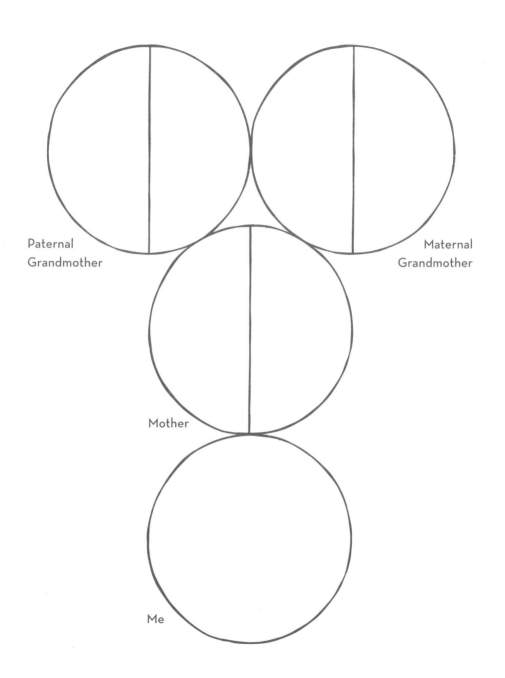

Paternal
Grandmother

Maternal
Grandmother

Mother

Me

In the previous exercise, what ended up in the circle of you as a mother? It's so easy to focus on what we don't want to pass on that we forget what we *do* want to pass on from our lineage. What are you determined to carry forward from your mother line?

• • • • •

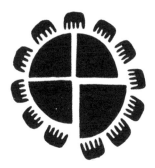

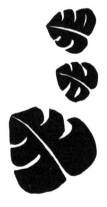

Imagine you are going to tell your child their birth story, without medical details, in an allegorical way. Draw or write a symbolic version of your birth story.

Here are some questions to guide your story:
If your birth were a landscape, what would the weather be like?
The terrain (forest, desert, ocean, etc.)? The path? What creatures would you encounter? What would the title be? (Remember that this is directed at your child, whose psyche is craving fairytale-like metaphors rather than literal details of a vacuum extraction or whatever else happened.)

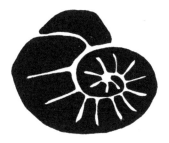

What has early motherhood taught you
that you couldn't have learned any other way?

• • • • •

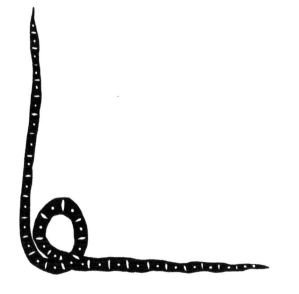

What is one ritual you definitely want to create
or maintain for your family?

· · · · ·

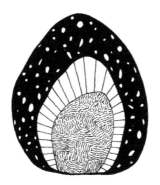

Write a letter to your child telling them what you most want them to know about their birth, or this postpartum time you've had together, and what you want them to know if they have children.

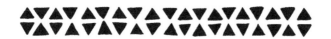

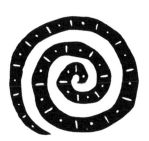

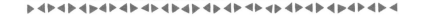

TRUST

Oh my child, lie back. Feel me.
I am the Grandmother's embrace.
The wide lap, deep bosom, smell of mother's milk.

Don't do this yourself.
Oh no, trust the dirt, the roots
beneath the dirt—
oh yes, those you cannot see.

Do you know what is in the space between the stars of Orion's belt?
Of course not, there are mysteries, my daughter.

You wear yourself out with the churning, rumbling,
back and forth, around and around.

Oh my friend,
Dive deeper.
Into the source of the source of the source
You cannot see. But you know her.

Lean into the unknowable, the unseeable, the unspeakable.
Revel in the hammock of the space
Between the stars of your favorite constellation.

Then when you've lain in Grandmother's lap,
On the dirt above sprawling roots,
And in celestial space,

Exhale again.

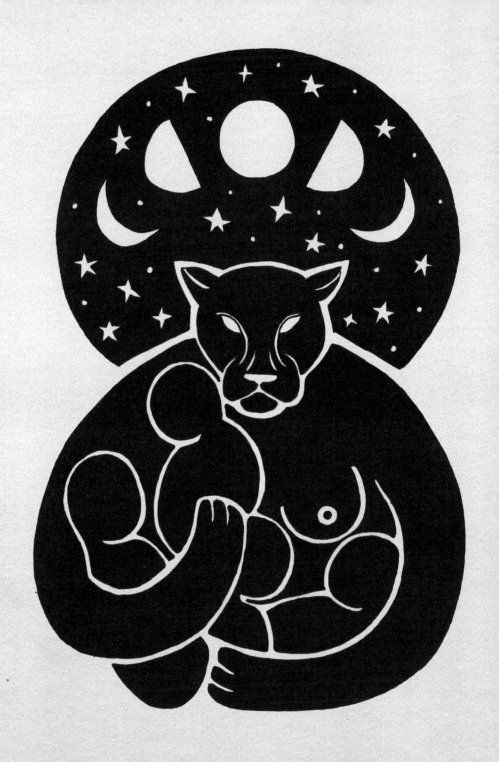

— With Thanks —

A circle of women came together to support the birth of this project. It was at the suggestion of my editor Beth Frankl that we continue the work of *The Fourth Trimester*, allowing it to evolve into more useful tools to support women into this journey of motherhood. Shambhala embraced my vision of moving away from the original beautiful watercolors from *The Fourth Trimester* book and card deck into the bolder archetypal work of Joanna Johnson, who created this work while in my MotherCircle class, long before this journal was conceived.. The organic nature and symbiosis of two single moms contending with race, creativity, artistry, and womanhood searching for what is true and whole in the journey was a thrill. It was a dream to bring forth the strength and gravitas of what becoming a mother means, as a shared vision. Jamie Mossay brought her birth story expertise and helped refine the questions, especially for MotherBaby and MotherBirth. Kristin Hauser, in the midst of her early mothering journey, gave feedback on the poignancy of the questions and also offered simple do-able practices for the beginning of some of the chapters. Ash Robinson came to the rescue while I was in the middle of two books at the same time to offer editing support, making sure I got to the finish line. Sil Reynolds and Liz Koch were my fairy godmothers, tracking the truth of my vision and holding me accountable to my own soul in the process. Val Matos created and maintained our nest, caring for both me and Cece while I wrote and created—she was my steadfast cheerleader and safety net. And to Maureen, Marilyn, Linda, and Kristine. All of these women are my many mothers.

Shambhala Publications, Inc.
4720 Walnut Street
Boulder, Colorado 80301
www.shambhala.com

Cover art: Joanna Johnson
Cover design: Allison Meierding
Interior design: Allison Meierding

9 8 7 6 5 4 3 2 1

First Edition
Printed in Singapore

Library of Congress Cataloging-in-Publication Data
Names: Johnson, Kimberly Ann, author.
Title: The fourth trimester journal: practices and reflections
to honor your journey into motherhood /
Kimberly Ann Johnson.
Description: First edition. | Boulder, Colorado:
Shambhala Publications, Inc., [2021]
Identifiers: LCCN 2020051531 | ISBN 9781611808384 (trade paperback)
Subjects: LCSH: Mothers—Diaries. | Mothers—Life skills guides. |
Mothers—Health and hygiene--Miscellanea. |
Mother and child—Miscellanea. | Diaries—Authorship.
Classification: LCC HQ759 .J64373 2021 | DDC 306.874/3—dc23
LC record available at https://lccn.loc.gov/2020051531